Mediterranean Diet for Everyone

Simple and Affordable Mediterranean Recipes to Start Managing Your Weight and Boost Your Lifestyle

America Best Recipes

Table of contents

Courgette, Fennel, and Orange Salad

Preparation Time: 15 minutes

Cooking Time: 0 minutes

Servings: 4

Ingredients :

- 1 orange
- 2 small courgettes (green or yellow)
- 2 small fennel bulbs
- 2 tsp. sherry vinegar
- 4 tbsp. olive oil
- 1 Baby Gem lettuce, washed and leaves separated
- Juice ½ lemon

Directions:

1. Cut the peel off the orange. Remove any pith. Slice the orange and halve each slice. Ideally, you should be cutting the orange on a plate or the chopping board since we are going to collect the juice left over from the cutting.

2. Take the fennel and remove any outer leaves that are tough. Cut the cores into halves and then slice them as thinly as you can.
3. Remove the ends of the courgettes and shave thin and long slices using a vegetable peeler. You can toss away the watery and seedy centers.
4. Take a small bowl and mix together olive oil, vinegar, and the orange juice left over on the plate or chopping board.
5. Take out another bowl and mix the courgette, fennel, orange slices, and lettuce leaves.
6. Serve the fennel mixture and top it with the orange juice dressing.

Nutrition:

Calories: 170 Calories

Protein: 3 g

Fat: 12 g

Carbs: 10 g

Potato Salad

Preparation Time: 10 minutes

Cooking Time: 6 minutes

Servings: 4

Ingredients :

- 1 small onion, thinly sliced
- 1 tbsp. olive oil
- 1 garlic clove, crushed
- 3.5 oz. roasted red pepper sliced
- 25 g black olive, sliced
- 1 tsp. fresh oregano
- 7 oz. canned cherry tomatoes
- 10 oz. new potato, halved if large
- Handful basil leaves, torn

Directions:

1. Take out a saucepan and place it over medium heat. Pour the olive oil into it and allow it to heat. Add the onions and cook for about 10 minutes, or until the onions have become soft.

2. Add oregano and garlic. Cook for another 1 minute.

3. Add the peppers and tomato. Let the mixture simmer for about 10 minutes.

4. Use a pan and place it over medium-high heat. Bring it to a boil and then add the potatoes into the water. Cook the potatoes for about 15 minutes, or until they turn tender. Drain the potatoes.

5. Take out a small bowl and add the pepper and tomato sauce into it. Toss in the potatoes and mix well.

6. Serve your salad with a sprinkle of basil and olives.

Nutrition:

Calories: 111 Calories

Protein: 3 g

Fat: 4 g

Carbs: 16 g

Tomato, Cucumber, and Feta Salad

Preparation Time: 10 minutes

Cooking Time: 0 minutes

Servings: 4

Ingredients :

- 3 tbsp. extra-virgin olive oil
- ½ tsp. Dijon mustard
- 4 medium Persian cucumbers, thinly sliced crosswise
- 1 tsp. chopped fresh oregano, plus extra for garnish
- 1 1/2 tbsp. red-wine vinegar
- 1 cup (8 oz.) tomatoes, cut into wedges
- 1/4 tsp. salt
- 1 1/2 oz. feta cheese, crumbled

Directions:

1. Take out a medium bowl and combine oregano, vinegar, mustard, and salt.
2. Drizzle the oil on top. Add tomatoes, cucumbers, and feta.
3. Mix them well and serve with oregano leaves toppings, if you prefer.
4. Refrigerate if you are planning to serve later.

Nutrition:

Calories: 153 Calories

Protein: 3 g

Fat: 13.1 g

Carbs: 6.1 g

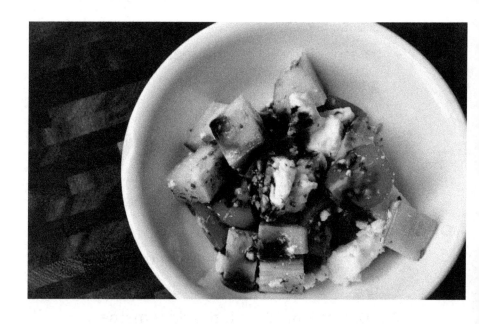

Goat Cheese Stuffed Tomatoes

Preparation Time: 10 minutes

Cooking Time: 6 minutes

Servings: 4

Ingredients:

- 6-8 arugula leaves
- 3 oz. crumbled feta cheese
- 2 medium ripe tomatoes
- Extra-virgin olive oil to drizzle
- Balsamic vinegar to drizzle
- 1 red onion, very thinly sliced for garnish
- Fresh chopped parsley for garnish
- Salt and freshly ground pepper to taste

Directions:

1. Arrange the arugula leaves in the center of a plate.
2. Remove the tops and the core of the tomatoes. Ideally, you should remove the top first and scoop out the core.
3. Fill the tomatoes with feta cheese. Add salt and pepper, to taste
4. Drizzle with olive oil and balsamic vinegar.
5. Garnish with chopped parsley and red onion.
6. Serve at room temperature.

Nutrition:

Calories: 142 Calories

Protein: 7 g

Fat: 13.1 g

Carbs: 7 g

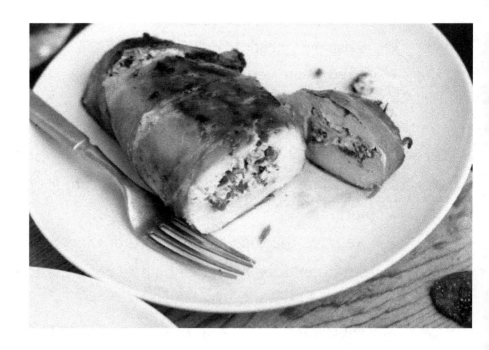

Classic Tabbouleh

Preparation Time: 10 minutes

Cooking Time: 10 minutes

Servings: 4

Ingredients :

- ¾ cup bulgur
- 2 cups freshly chopped parsley
- 1½ cups water
- ½ cup fresh lemon juice
- ½ cup extra-virgin olive oil
- ½ red bell pepper, diced
- 3 ripe plum tomatoes, peeled, seeded, and diced
- 1 large cucumber, peeled, seeded, and diced
- ¾ cup chopped scallions, white and green parts
- ½ green bell pepper, diced
- ½ cup finely chopped fresh mint
- Handful of greens for serving
- Seasoned pita wedges
- Sea salt and freshly ground pepper to taste

Directions:

1. Preheat the oven to around 375°F.
2. Take a medium-sized bowl and add the asparagus with 2 tbsp. of salt and olive oil.
3. Take out a baking dish and add the asparagus. Place the tray in the oven and roast for about 10 minutes, or until the asparagus becomes tender.
4. Take out the asparagus and set aside.
5. Use another medium-sized bowl and add garlic, lime juice, orange juice, and remaining 2 tbsp. of olive oil. Whisk all the ingredients together. Add salt and pepper to taste.
6. Take the lettuce and split it into 6 plates. Take out the asparagus and place it on top of the lettuce.
7. Pour the dressing over the asparagus and lettuce salad. Top the salad with basil and pine nuts. Add a small amount of Romano cheese for garnish, if you prefer.
8. You can also toast the pine nuts in the oven. Use the method below:

9.   Take out a baking tray and line it with a non-stick baking sheet. Add the pine nuts on top.

10.   Bake at 375°F for about 5-10 minutes, or until the nuts are lightly browned.

11.   Remove from the oven and set aside to cool.

12.   Add the nuts to the salad as a topping.

Nutrition:

Calories: 177 Calories

Protein: 12 g

Fat: 11 g

Carbs: 28 g

Mediterranean Greens

Preparation Time: 10 minutes

Cooking Time: 0 minutes

Servings: 4

Ingredients :

- 6 cups assorted fresh mixed greens (such as radicchio, arugula, watercress, baby spinach, and romaine)
- 1 small red onion, thinly sliced
- 20 cherry tomatoes, halved
- ¼ cup dried cranberries
- ¼ cup chopped walnuts
- Crumbled feta cheese
- Freshly ground pepper to taste
- 2 tbsp. balsamic vinegar
- 2 cloves fresh garlic, finely minced
- 4 tbsp. extra-virgin olive oil
- 1 tbsp. water
- ½ tsp. crushed dried oregano

Directions:

1. Take out a large salad bowl, combine walnuts, greens, tomatoes, onion, and cranberries. Gently toss.
2. For the dressing, combine water, vinegar, oregano, olive oil, and garlic. Mix the ingredients well. Pour over the salad and lightly toss.
3. Add feta cheese as garnish, if preferred.
4. Add pepper to taste.

Nutrition:

Calories: 140 Calories

Protein: 2 g

Fat: 12 g

Carbs: 6 g

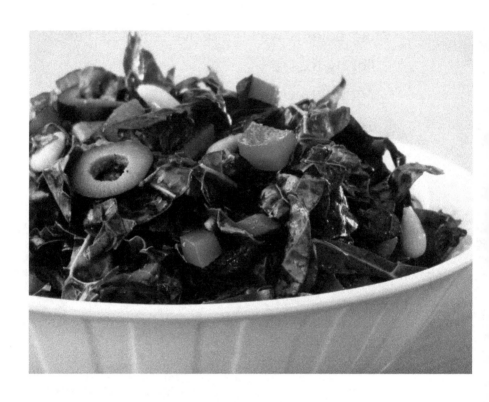

Classic Greek Salad

Preparation Time: 15 minutes

Cooking Time: 0 minutes

Servings: 6

Ingredients:

- 6 large firm tomatoes, quartered
- 20 Greek black olives
- ½ lb. Greek feta cheese, cut into small cubes
- ½ head of escarole, shredded
- 3 tbsp. red wine vinegar
- ¼ cup extra-virgin olive oil
- 1 tbsp. dried oregano
- ½ English cucumber, peeled, seeded, and thinly sliced
- 2 cloves fresh garlic, finely minced
- ½ red onion, sliced
- 1 medium red bell pepper, seeded and sliced
- ¼ cup freshly chopped Italian parsley
- Salt and freshly ground pepper to taste

Directions:

1. Take out a large bowl and add vinegar, oregano, olive oil, and garlic. Add salt and pepper to taste. Set aside the bowl.
2. In another large bowl, add onion, tomatoes, escarole, cucumber, bell pepper, and cheese and mix them well.
3. Take the vinegar mixture and pour it over the salad in the second bowl.
4. Top the salad with olives and parsley.

Nutrition:

Calories: 268 Calories

Protein: 23 g

Fat: 17 g

Carbs: 44 g

North African Zucchini Salad

Preparation Time: 10 minutes

Cooking Time: 0 minutes

Servings: 4

Ingredients :

- 1 lb. firm green zucchini, thinly sliced
- ½ tsp. ground cumin
- 2 cloves fresh garlic, finely minced
- Juice from 1 large lemon
- 1 tbsp. extra-virgin olive oil
- 1½ tbsp. plain low-fat yogurt
- Crumbled feta cheese
- Finely chopped parsley for garnish
- Salt and freshly ground pepper to taste

Directions:

1. Add the zucchini into a large saucepan and steam it for about 2-5 minutes, or until it becomes tender and crispy. Place the zucchini under cold water and drain well.

21

2. Take out a large bowl and mix cumin, olive oil, lemon juice, garlic, and yogurt. Add salt and pepper to taste.

3. Add the zucchini into the mixture in the bowl and toss gently.

4. Serve with feta cheese and parsley as garnish.

Nutrition:

Calories: 140 Calories

Protein: 2 g

Fat: 12 g

Carbs: 6 g

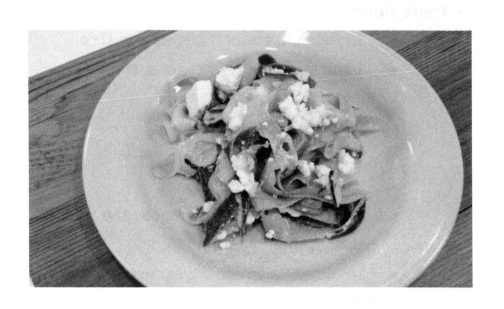

Tunisian Style Carrot Salad

Preparation Time: 15 minutes

Cooking Time: 0 minutes

Servings: 6

Ingredients :

- 10 medium carrots, peeled and sliced
- 1 cup crumbled feta cheese, divided
- 2 tsp. caraway seed
- ¼ cup extra-virgin olive oil
- 6 tbsp. apple cider vinegar
- 5 tsp. freshly minced garlic
- 1 tbsp. Harissa paste (choose the level of heat based on your preference)
- 20 pitted Kalamata olives, reserving some for garnish
- Salt to taste

Directions:

1. Take out a medium saucepan and place it on medium heat. Fill it with water and add the carrots. Cook carrots until tender. Drain and cool the carrots under cold water. Drain again to remove any excess water.

24

2. Take out a large bowl and place the carrots in them.

3. Take out a mortar and combine salt, garlic, and caraway seeds. Grind them until they form a paste. Otherwise, you can also use a small bowl, preferably one not made out of glass for grind. The final option would be to toss the ingredients into a blender and pulse them.

4. Add vinegar and Harissa into the bowl with the carrots and mix them well.

5. Use a large spoon and mash the carrots. Add the garlic mixture into the carrot and mix again until they have all blended well. Add the olive oil and mix again.

6. Finally, add about ½ the feta cheese and all the olives and mix well again.

7. Take out a large bowl and add the salad to it. Top it with the remaining feta cheese.

Nutrition:

Calories: 138 Calories

Protein: 7 g

Fat: 5 g

Carbs: 13 g

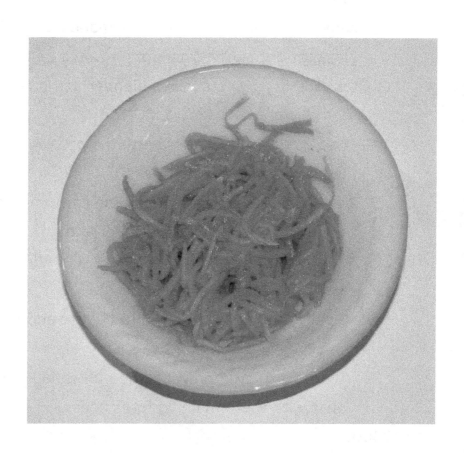

Caesar Salad

Preparation Time: 5 minutes

Cooking Time: 0 minutes

Servings: 6

Ingredients:

- 10 small pitted black olives, chopped
- 1-2 bunches romaine lettuce, cleaned and torn in pieces
- 2 tsp. lemon juice
- 2½ tsp. balsamic vinegar
- ½ cup grated parmesan cheese
- ½ cup nonfat plain yogurt
- 1 tsp. worcestershire sauce
- ½ tsp. anchovy paste
- 2 cloves freshly minced garlic

Directions:

1. Take out a large bowl and place romaine lettuce in it.

2. Take out your blended and add mix lemon juice, yogurt, garlic, anchovy paste, vinegar, worcestershire sauce, and ¼ cup parmesan cheese. Mix all the ingredients well until they are smooth.
3. Pour the yogurt mixture over the lettuce and toss lightly.
4. Top the salad with the remaining parmesan cheese.

Nutrition:

Calories: 49 Calories

Protein: 4 g

Fat: 1 g

Carbs: 4 g

Avocado Salad

Preparation Time: 10 minutes

Cooking Time: 0 minutes

Servings: 3

Ingredients :

- 1 small onion, finely chopped
- 1 large ripe avocado, pitted and peeled
- 2 tbsp. chopped fresh parsley
- 2 tsp. fresh lime juice
- ½ small hot pepper, finely chopped (optional)
- 1 cup halved cherry tomatoes
- Salt and freshly ground pepper to taste

Directions:

1. Start with the avocado and cut it into bite-sized pieces.
2. Add parsley, lime juice, tomatoes, onion, and hot pepper. Mix all the ingredients well. Add salt and pepper to taste.
3. Finally, add the avocado into the mixture and mix them well.

Nutrition:

Calories: 130 Calories

Protein: 2 g

Fat: 10 g

Carbs: 10 g

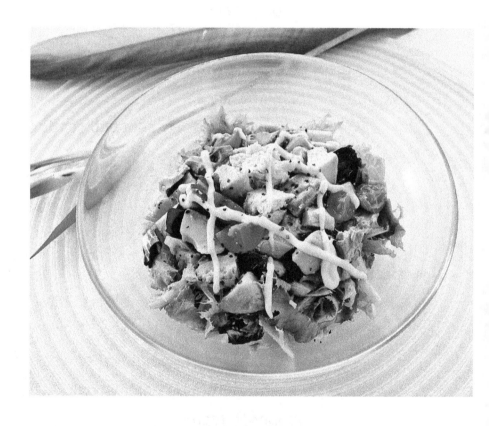

Spanish Salad

Preparation Time: 10 minutes

Cooking Time: 0 minutes

Servings: 6

Ingredients :

- 2 bunches romaine lettuce, cleaned and trimmed
- 1 large sweet onion, thinly sliced
- 3 medium ripe tomatoes, chopped
- 3 tbsp. balsamic vinegar
- ¼ cup extra-virgin olive oil
- 1 red bell pepper, seeded and thinly sliced
- 1 green bell pepper, seeded and thinly sliced
- ¼ cup chopped and pitted black olives
- ¼ cup chopped and pitted marinated green olives
- Salt and freshly ground pepper to taste

Directions:

1. Take out 6 plates and place romaine lettuce on them to form a base.
2. Add peppers, tomatoes, onion, and olives on top of each of the lettuce bases.
3. In a small bowl, combine olive oil and vinegar together. Add the dressing over the salad.
4. Add salt and pepper to taste, if preferred.

Nutrition:

Calories: 107 Calories

Protein: 2 g

Fat: 9 g

Carbs: 6 g

Parsley Couscous Salad

Preparation Time: 2 hours

Cooking Time: 0 minutes

Servings: 4

Ingredients :

- ¼ cup couscous
- 2 tsp. extra-virgin olive oil
- ¼ cup water
- 2 tsp. lemon zest
- 1 medium ripe tomato, peeled, seeded, and diced
- 2 tbsp. pine nuts
- 2 tbsp. fresh lemon juice
- ¼ cup finely chopped fresh flat parsley leaves
- 2 tbsp. finely chopped fresh mint leaves
- 2 heads Belgian endive, leaves for scooping
- Whole wheat pita rounds, cut into wedges and toasted until crispy
- Salt and freshly ground pepper to taste

Directions:

1. Take out a medium bowl and then combine lemon juice and water. All the mixture to stand for about 1 hour.

2. After the hour, add mint, parsley, lemon zest, olive oil, and pine nuts. Mix the ingredients well.

3. Add in the couscous to the mixture. Allow it to stand for about 1 hour. After 1 hour, add salt and pepper to taste.

4. Place couscous mixture in the center of a plate and top it with tomato. You can surround the couscous salad with toasted pita wedges and endive leaves, which makes for a wonderful presentation.

5. Refrigerator overnight so that you can have it the next day.

Nutrition:

Calories: 120 Calories

Protein: 5 g

Fat: 2 g

Carbs: 18 g

Cress and Tangerine Salad

Preparation Time: 15 minutes

Cooking Time: 0 minutes

Servings: 4

Ingredients :

- 4 large sweet tangerines
- ¼ cup extra-virgin olive oil
- 2 large bunches watercress, washed and stems removed
- Juice from 1 fresh lemon
- 10 cherry tomatoes, halved
- 16 pitted Kalamata olives
- Sea salt and freshly ground pepper to taste

Directions:

1. Take the tangerines and peel them into a medium-sized bowl. Make sure that you remove any pits and squeeze the sections. You should have around ¼ cup of tangerine juice. Set sections aside.

2. Take a large bowl and add lemon juice, tangerine juice, and olive oil. Mix them together and add salt and pepper for flavor, if you prefer.
3. Use paper towels to pat the cress dry. Add watercress, tomatoes, and olives to the bowl containing the tangerine sections (not to be confused with the bowl containing tangerine juice). Toss them lightly.
4. Pour the tangerine juice mixture on top. Mix well and serve.

Nutrition:

Calories: 195 Calories

Protein: 3 g

Fat: 16 g

Carbs: 14 g

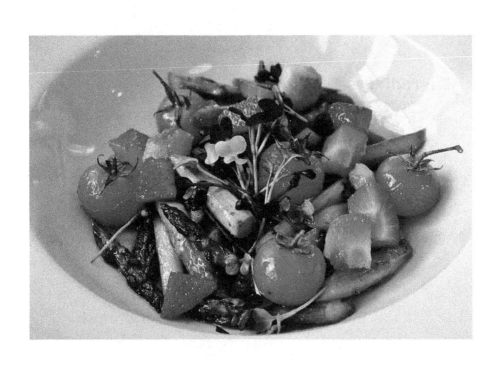

Prosciutto and Figs Salad

Preparation Time: 10 minutes

Cooking Time: 0 minutes

Servings: 4

Ingredients :

- One 10-12-oz. package fresh baby spinach
- 1 small hot red chili pepper, finely diced
- 1 carton figs, stems removed and quartered
- ½ cup walnuts, coarsely chopped
- 1 tbsp. fresh orange juice
- 1 tbsp. honey
- 4 slices prosciutto, cut into strips
- Shaved parmesan cheese for garnish

Directions:

1. Take your spinach and divide them into 4 equal portions. Each portion should be on a separate plate and will act as a base. Add

quartered prosciutto, figs, and walnuts on each spinach as toppings.

2.   For the dressing, take a small bowl and add honey, orange juice, and diced pepper. Add the mixture over the salad.

3.   Finally, toss the salad lightly and use parmesan cheese for the garnish.

Nutrition:

Calories: 190 Calories

Protein: 26 g

Fat: 9 g

Carbs: 17 g

Garden Vegetables and Chickpeas Salad

Preparation Time: 10 minutes

Cooking Time: 0 minutes

Servings: 4

Ingredients :

- 2 tbsp. freshly squeezed lemon juice
- 1/8 tsp. freshly ground pepper
- 1 cup cubed part-skim mozzarella cheese
- 1 tbsp. fresh basil leaf, snipped
- 1 (15-oz.) can chickpeas, rinsed and well drained
- 2 cups coarsely chopped fresh broccoli
- 2 cloves fresh garlic, finely minced
- ½ cup sliced fresh carrots
- 1 7½-oz. can diced tomatoes, undrained

Directions:

1. Use a large bowl and add garlic, basil, lemon juice, and ground pepper. Mix them well.
2. Add the chickpeas, carrots, tomatoes with juice, broccoli, and mozzarella cheese. Toos all the ingredients well.
3. You can serve immediately, or you can keep it refrigerated overnight.

Nutrition:

Calories: 195 Calories

Protein: 16 g

Fat: 7 g

Carbs: 24 g

Peppered Watercress Salad

Preparation Time: 5 minutes

Cooking Time: 0 minutes

Servings: 4

Ingredients :

- 2 tsp. champagne vinegar
- 2 bunches (about 8 cups) watercress, rinsed and rough stems removed
- 2 tbsp. extra-virgin olive oil
- Salt and freshly ground pepper to taste

Directions:

1. Drain the watercress properly.
2. Take out a small bowl and then add salt, pepper, vinegar, and olive oil. Mix them well together.
3. Transfer the watercress to a bowl. Add the vinegar mixture into it and toss well.
4. Serve immediately.

Nutrition:

Calories: 67 Calories

Protein: 4 g

Fat: 7 g

Carbs: 1 g

Rustic Vegetable and Brown Rice Bowl

Preparation Time: 15 minutes

Cooking Time: 10 minutes

Servings: 4

Ingredients :

- Nonstick cooking spray
- 2 cups broccoli florets
- 2 cups cauliflower florets
- 1 (15-oz.) can chickpeas, drained and rinsed
- 1 cup carrots sliced 1 inch thick
- 2 to 3 tbsp. extra-virgin olive oil, divided
- Salt and freshly ground black pepper
- 2 to 3 tbsp. sesame seeds, for garnish
- 2 cups cooked brown rice

For the dressing

- 3 to 4 tbsp. tahini
- 2 tbsp. honey
- 1 lemon, juiced
- 1 garlic clove, minced
- Salt
- Freshly ground black pepper

Directions:

1. Preheat the oven to 400°F. Spray two baking sheets with cooking spray.
2. Cover the first baking sheet with the broccoli and cauliflower and the second with the chickpeas and carrots. Toss each sheet with half of the oil and season with salt and pepper before placing in oven.
3. Cook the carrots and chickpeas for 10 minutes, leaving the carrots still just crisp, and the broccoli and cauliflower for 20 minutes, until tender. Stir each halfway through cooking.
4. To make the dressing, in a small bowl, mix the tahini, honey, lemon juice, and garlic. Season with salt and pepper and set aside.
5. Divide the rice into individual bowls, then layer with vegetables and drizzle dressing over the dish.

Nutrition:

Calories: 192;

Carbs: 12.7g;

Protein: 3.8g;

Fat: 15.5g

Roasted Brussels sprouts And Pecans

Preparation Time: 10 minutes

Cooking Time: 15 minute

Servings: 4

Ingredients :

- 1 ½ lb. fresh Brussels sprouts
- 4 tbsp. olive oil
- 4 cloves of garlic, minced
- 3 tbsp. water
- Salt and pepper to taste
- ½ cup chopped pecans

Directions:

1. Place all ingredients in the Instant Pot.
2. Combine all ingredients until well combined.
3. Close the lid and make sure that the steam release vent is set to "Venting."
4. Press the "Slow Cook" button and adjust the cooking time to 3 hours.
5. Sprinkle with a dash of lemon juice if desired.

Nutrition:

Calories: 161;

Carbs: 10.2g;

Protein: 4.1g;

Fat: 13.1g

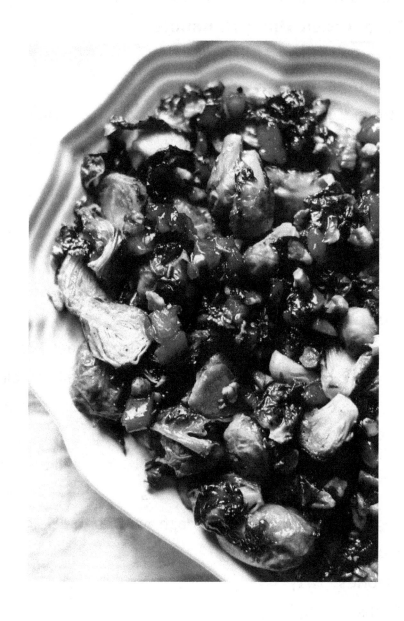

Eggs with Zucchini Noodles

Preparation Time: 10 minutes

Cooking Time: 11 minutes

Servings: 2

Ingredients:

- 2 tbsp. extra-virgin olive oil
- 3 zucchinis, cut with a spiralizer
- 4 eggs
- Salt and black pepper to the taste
- A pinch of red pepper flakes
- Cooking spray
- 1 tbsp. basil, chopped

Directions:

1. In a bowl, combine the zucchini noodles with salt, pepper and the olive oil and toss well.
2. Grease a baking sheet with cooking spray and divide the zucchini noodles into 4 nests on it.
3. Crack an egg on top of each nest, sprinkle salt, pepper and the pepper flakes on top and bake at 350°F for 11 minutes.
4. Divide the mix between plates, sprinkle the basil on top and serve.

Nutrition:

Calories 296,

Fat 23.6,

Fiber 3.3,

Carbs 10.6,

Protein 14.7

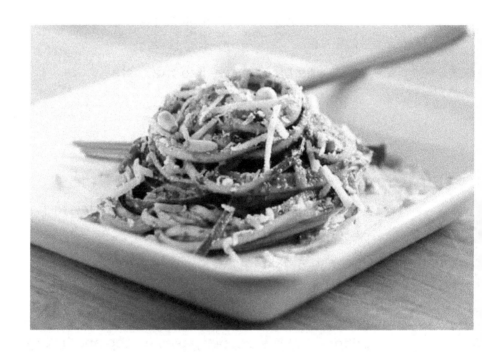

Roasted Root Veggies

Preparation Time: 20 minutes

Cooking Time: 1 hour 30 minute

Servings: 6

Ingredients :

- 2 tbsp. olive oil
- 1 head garlic, cloves separated and peeled
- 1 large turnip, peeled and cut into ½-inch pieces
- 1 medium sized red onion, cut into ½-inch pieces
- 1 ½ lbs. beets, trimmed but not peeled, scrubbed and cut into ½-inch pieces
- 1 ½ lbs. Yukon gold potatoes, unpeeled, cut into ½-inch pieces
- 2 ½ lbs. butternut squash, peeled, seeded, cut into ½-inch pieces

Directions:

1. Grease 2 rimmed and large baking sheets. Preheat oven to 425oF.
2. In a large bowl, mix all ingredients thoroughly.
3. Into the two baking sheets, evenly divide the root vegetables, spread in one layer.
4. Season generously with pepper and salt.
5. Pop into the oven and roast for 1 hour and 15 minute or until golden brown and tender.
6. Remove from oven and let it cool for at least 15 minutes before serving.

Nutrition:

Calories: 298;

Carbs: 61.1g;

Protein: 7.4g;

Fat: 5.0g

Roasted Vegetables and Zucchini Pasta

Preparation Time: 10 minutes

Cooking Time: 7 minute

Servings: 2

Ingredients :

- ¼ cup raw pine nuts
- 4 cups leftover vegetables
- 2 garlic cloves, minced
- 1 tbsp. extra virgin olive oil
- 4 medium zucchinis, cut into long strips resembling noodles

Directions:

1. Heat oil in a large skillet over medium heat and sauté the garlic for 2 minutes.
2. Add the leftover vegetables and place the zucchini noodles on top. Let it cook for five minutes. Garnish with pine nuts.

Nutrition:

Calories: 288;

Carbs: 23.6g;

Protein: 8.2g;

Fat: 19.2g

Sautéed Collard Greens

Preparation Time: 10 minutes

Cooking Time: 0 minute

Servings: 4

Ingredients :

- 1-lb. fresh collard greens, cut into 2-inch pieces
- 1 pinch red pepper flakes
- 3 cups chicken broth
- 1 tsp. pepper
- 1 tsp. salt
- 2 cloves garlic, minced
- 1 large onion, chopped
- 3 slices bacon
- 1 tbsp. olive oil

Directions:

1. Using a large skillet, heat oil on medium-high heat. Sauté bacon until crisp. Remove it from

the pan and crumble it once cooled. Set it aside.

2. Using the same pan, sauté onion and cook until tender. Add garlic until fragrant. Add the collard greens and cook until they start to wilt.
3. Pour in the chicken broth and season with pepper, salt and red pepper flakes. Reduce the heat to low and simmer for 45 minutes.

Nutrition:

Calories: 20;

Carbs: 3.0g;

Protein: 1.0g;

Fat: 1.0g

Savoy Cabbage with Coconut Cream Sauce

Preparation Time: 5 minutes

Cooking Time: 20 minute

Servings: 4

Ingredients :

- 3 tbsp. olive oil
- 1 onion, chopped
- 4 cloves of garlic, minced
- 1 head savoy cabbage, chopped finely
- 2 cups bone broth
- 1 cup coconut milk, freshly squeezed
- 1 bay leaf
- Salt and pepper to taste
- 2 tbsp. chopped parsley

Directions:

1. Heat oil in a pot for 2 minutes.
2. Stir in the onions, bay leaf, and garlic until fragrant, around 3 minutes.
3. Add the rest of the ingredients, except for the parsley and mix well.
4. Cover pot, bring to a boil, and let it simmer for 5 minutes or until cabbage is tender to taste.
5. Stir in parsley and serve.

Nutrition:

Calories: 195;

Carbs: 12.3g;

Protein: 2.7g;

Fat: 19.7g

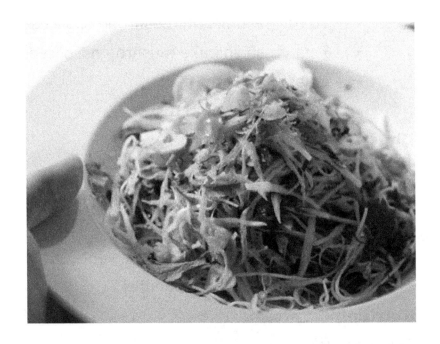

Slow Cooked Buttery Mushrooms

Preparation Time: 10 minutes

Cooking Time: 10 minute

Servings: 2

Ingredients :

- 2 tbsp. butter
- 2 tbsp. olive oil
- 3 cloves of garlic, minced
- 16 oz. fresh brown mushrooms, sliced
- 7 oz. fresh shiitake mushrooms, sliced
- A dash of thyme
- Salt and pepper to taste

Directions:

1. Heat the butter and oil in a pot.
2. Sauté the garlic until fragrant, around 1 minute.
3. Stir in the rest of the ingredients and cook until soft, around 9 minutes.

Nutrition:

Calories: 192;

Carbs: 12.7g;

Protein: 3.8g;

Fat: 15.5g

Steamed Squash Chowder

Preparation Time: 20 minutes

Cooking Time: 40 minute

Servings: 4

Ingredients :

- 3 cups chicken broth
- 2 tbsp. ghee
- 1 tsp. chili powder
- ½ tsp. cumin
- 1 ½ tsp. salt
- 2 tsp. cinnamon
- 3 tbsp. olive oil
- 2 carrots, chopped
- 1 small yellow onion, chopped
- 1 green apple, sliced and cored
- 1 large butternut squash, peeled, seeded, and chopped to ½-inch cubes

Directions:

1. In a large pot on medium high fire, melt ghee.
2. Once ghee is hot, sauté onions for 5 minutes or until soft and translucent.
3. Add olive oil, chili powder, cumin, salt, and cinnamon. Sauté for half a minute.
4. Add chopped squash and apples.
5. Sauté for 10 minutes while stirring once in a while.
6. Add broth, cover and cook on medium fire for twenty minutes or until apples and squash are tender.
7. With an immersion blender, puree chowder. Adjust consistency by adding more water.
8. Add more salt or pepper depending on desire.
9. Serve and enjoy.

Nutrition:

Calories: 228;

Carbs: 17.9g;

Protein: 2.2g;

Fat: 18.0g

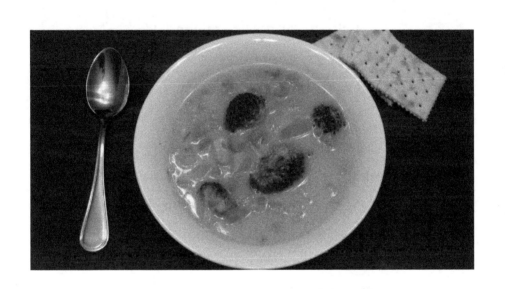

Steamed Zucchini-Paprika

Preparation Time: 15 minutes

Cooking Time: 30 minute

Servings: 2

Ingredients :

- 4 tbsp. olive oil
- 3 cloves of garlic, minced
- 1 onion, chopped
- 3 medium-sized zucchinis, sliced thinly
- A dash of paprika
- Salt and pepper to taste

Directions:

1. Place all ingredients in the Instant Pot.
2. Give a good stir to combine all ingredients.
3. Close the lid and make sure that the steam release valve is set to "Venting."
4. Press the "Slow Cook" button and adjust the cooking time to 4 hours.
5. Halfway through the cooking time, open the lid and give a good stir to brown the other side.

Nutrition:

Calories: 93;

Carbs: 3.1g;

Protein: 0.6g;

Fat: 10.2g

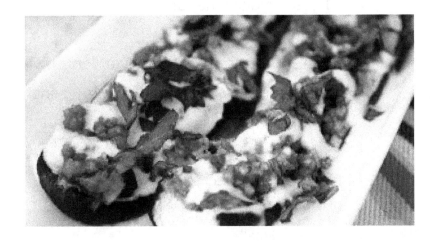

Stir Fried Brussels sprouts and Carrots

Preparation Time: 10 minutes

Cooking Time: 15 minute

Servings: 6

Ingredients :

- 1 tbsp. cider vinegar
- 1/3 cup water
- 1 lb. Brussels sprouts, halved lengthwise
- 1 lb. carrots cut diagonally into ½-inch thick lengths
- 3 tbsp. unsalted butter, divided
- 2 tbsp. chopped shallot
- ½ tsp. pepper
- ¾ tsp. salt

Directions:

1. On medium high fire, place a nonstick medium fry pan and heat 2 tbsp. butter.

2.   Add shallots and cook until softened, around one to two minutes while occasionally stirring.

3.   Add pepper salt, Brussels sprouts and carrots. Stir fry until vegetables starts to brown on the edges, around 3 to 4 minutes.

4.   Add water, cook and cover.

5.   After 5 to 8 minutes, or when veggies are already soft, add remaining butter.

6.   If needed season with more pepper and salt to taste.

7.   Turn off fire, transfer to a platter, serve and enjoy.

Nutrition:

Calories: 98;

Carbs: 13.9g;

Protein: 3.5g;

Fat: 4.2g

Stir Fried Eggplant

Preparation Time: 10 minutes

Cooking Time: 30 minute

Servings: 2

Ingredients :

- 1 tsp. cornstarch + 2 tbsp. water, mixed
- 1 tsp. brown sugar
- 2 tbsp. oyster sauce
- 1 tbsp. fish sauce
- 2 tbsp. soy sauce
- ½ cup fresh basil
- 2 tbsp. oil
- ¼ cup water
- 2 cups Chinese eggplant, spiral
- 1 red chili
- 6 cloves garlic, minced
- ½ purple onion, sliced thinly
- 1 3-oz package medium firm tofu, cut into slivers

Directions:

1. Prepare sauce by mixing cornstarch and water in a small bowl. In another bowl mix brown sugar, oyster sauce and fish sauce and set aside.

2. On medium high fire, place a large nonstick saucepan and heat 2 tbsp. oil. Sauté chili, garlic and onion for 4 minutes. Add tofu, stir fry for 4 minutes.

3. Add eggplant noodles and stir fry for 10 minutes. If pan dries up, add water in small amounts to moisten pan and cook noodles.

4. Pour in sauce and mix well. Once simmering, slowly add cornstarch mixer while continuing to mix vigorously. Once sauce thickens add fresh basil and cook for a minute.

5. Remove from fire, transfer to a serving plate and enjoy.

Nutrition:

Calories: 369;

Carbs: 28.4g;

Protein: 11.4g;

Fat: 25.3g

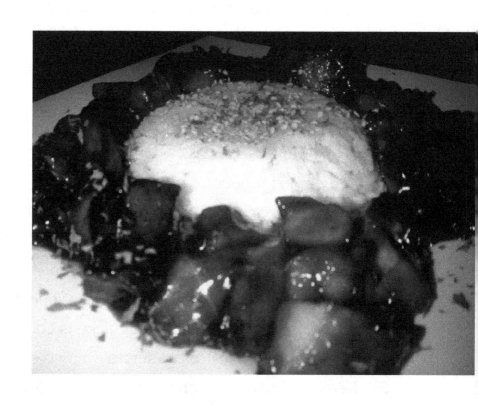

Summer Vegetables

Preparation Time: 20 minutes

Cooking Time: 1 hour 40 minutes minute

Servings: 6

Ingredients :

- 1 tsp. dried marjoram
- 1/3 cup Parmesan cheese
- 1 small eggplant, sliced into ¼-inch thick circles
- 1 small summer squash, peeled and sliced diagonally into ¼-inch thickness
- 3 large tomatoes, sliced into ¼-inch thick circles
- ½ cup dry white wine
- ½ tsp. freshly ground pepper, divided
- ½ tsp. salt, divided
- 5 cloves garlic, sliced thinly
- 2 cups leeks, sliced thinly
- 4 tbsp. extra virgin olive oil, divided

Directions:

1. On medium fire, place a large nonstick saucepan and heat 2 tbsp. oil.

2. Sauté garlic and leeks for 6 minutes or until garlic is starting to brown. Season with pepper and salt, ¼ tsp. each.

3. Pour in wine and cook for another minute. Transfer to a 2-quart baking dish.

4. In baking dish, layer in alternating pattern the eggplant, summer squash, and tomatoes. Do this until dish is covered with vegetables. If there are excess vegetables, store for future use.

5. Season with remaining pepper and salt. Drizzle with remaining olive oil and pop in a preheated 425oF oven.

6. Bake for 75 minutes. Remove from oven and top with marjoram and cheese.

7. Return to oven and bake for 15 minutes more or until veggies are soft and edges are browned.

8. Allow to cool for at least 5 minutes before serving.

Nutrition:

Calories: 150;

Carbs: 11.8g;

Protein: 3.3g;

Fat: 10.8g

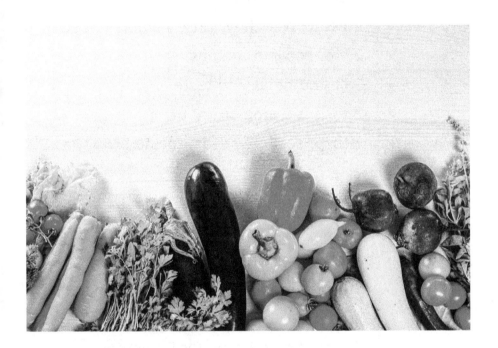

Stir Fried Bok Choy

Preparation Time: 5 minutes

Cooking Time: 13 minute

Servings: 4

Ingredients :

- 3 tbsp. coconut oil
- 4 cloves of garlic, minced
- 1 onion, chopped
- 2 heads bok choy, rinsed and chopped
- 2 tsp. coconut aminos
- Salt and pepper to taste
- 2 tbsp. sesame oil
- 2 tbsp. sesame seeds, toasted

Directions:

1. Heat the oil in a pot for 2 minutes.
2. Sauté the garlic and onions until fragrant, around 3 minutes.
3. Stir in the bok choy, coconut aminos, salt and pepper.
4. Cover pan and cook for 5 minutes.
5. Stir and continue cooking for another 3 minutes.
6. Drizzle with sesame oil and sesame seeds on top before serving.

Nutrition:

Calories: 358;

Carbs: 5.2g;

Protein: 21.5g;

Fat: 28.4g

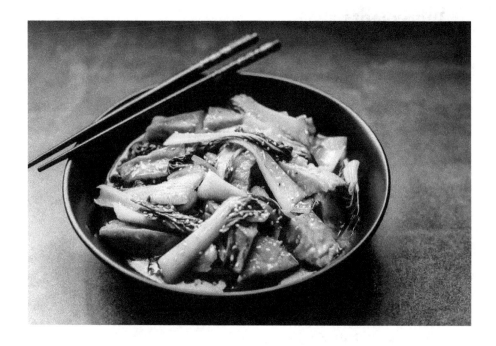

Summer Veggies in Instant Pot

Preparation Time: 10 minutes

Cooking Time: 7 minute

Servings: 6

Ingredients :

- 2 cups okra, sliced
- 1 cup grape tomatoes
- 1 cup mushroom, sliced
- 1 ½ cups onion, sliced
- 2 cups bell pepper, sliced
- 2 ½ cups zucchini, sliced
- 2 tbsp. basil, chopped
- 1 tbsp. thyme, chopped
- ½ cups balsamic vinegar
- ½ cups olive oil
- Salt and pepper

Directions:

1. Place all ingredients in the Instant Pot.
2. Stir the contents and close the lid.
3. Close the lid and press the Manual button.
4. Adjust the cooking time to 7 minutes.
5. Do quick pressure release.
6. Once cooled, evenly divide into serving size, keep in your preferred container, and refrigerate until ready to eat.

Nutrition:

Calories 233;

Carbs: 7g;

Protein: 3g;

Fat: 18g

Sumptuous Tomato Soup

Preparation Time: 10 minutes

Cooking Time: 30 minute

Servings: 2

Ingredients :

- Pepper and salt to taste
- 2 tbsp. tomato paste
- 1 ½ cups vegetable broth
- 1 tbsp. chopped parsley
- 1 tbsp. olive oil
- 5 garlic cloves
- ½ medium yellow onion
- 4 large ripe tomatoes

Directions:

1. Preheat oven to 350°F.
2. Chop onion and tomatoes into thin wedges. Place on a rimmed baking sheet. Season with parsley, pepper, salt, and olive oil. Toss to

combine well. Hide the garlic cloves inside tomatoes to keep it from burning.

3. Pop in the oven and bake for 30 minutes.
4. On medium pot, bring vegetable stock to a simmer. Add tomato paste.
5. Pour baked tomato mixture into pot. Continue simmering for another 10 minutes.
6. With an immersion blender, puree soup.
7. Adjust salt and pepper to taste before serving.

Nutrition:

Calories: 179;

Carbs: 26.7g;

Protein: 5.2g;

Fat: 7.7g

Superfast Cajun Asparagus

Preparation Time: 10 minutes

Cooking Time: 8 minute

Servings: 2

Ingredients :

- 1 tsp. Cajun seasoning
- 1-lb. asparagus
- 1 tsp. Olive oil

Directions:

1. Snap the asparagus and make sure that you use the tender part of the vegetable.
2. Place a large skillet on stovetop and heat on high for a minute.
3. Then grease skillet with cooking spray and spread asparagus in one layer.
4. Cover skillet and continue cooking on high for 5 to eight minutes.
5. Halfway through cooking time, stir skillet and then cover and continue to cook.

6. Once done cooking, transfer to plates, serve, and enjoy!

Nutrition:

Calories: 81;

Carbs: 0g;

Protein: 0g;

Fat: 9g

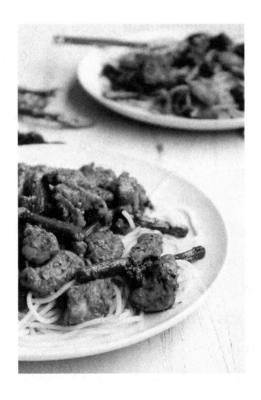

Sweet and Nutritious Pumpkin Soup

Preparation Time: 20 minutes

Cooking Time: 40 minute

Servings: 8

Ingredients :

- 1 tsp. chopped fresh parsley
- ½ cup half and half
- ½ tsp. chopped fresh thyme
- 1 tsp. salt
- 4 cups pumpkin puree
- 6 cups vegetable stock, divided
- 1 clove garlic, minced
- 1 1-inch piece gingerroot, peeled and minced
- 1 cup chopped onion

Directions:

1. On medium high fire, place a heavy bottomed pot and for 5 minutes heat ½ cup vegetable stock, ginger, garlic and onions or until veggies are tender.

2. Add remaining stock and cook for 30 minutes.

3. Season with thyme and salt.

4. With an immersion blender, puree soup until smooth.

5. Turn off fire and mix in half and half.

6. Transfer pumpkin soup into 8 bowls, garnish with parsley, serve and enjoy.

Nutrition:

Calories: 58;

Carbs: 6.6g;

Protein: 5.1g;

Fat: 1.7g

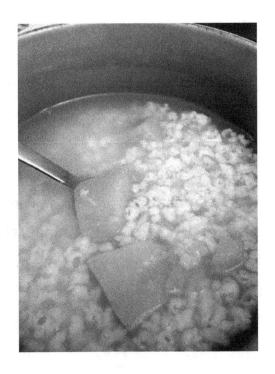

Sweet Potato Puree

Preparation Time: 10 minutes

Cooking Time: 15 minute

Servings: 6

Ingredients :

- 2 lb. sweet potatoes, peeled
- 1 ½ cups water
- 5 Medjool dates, pitted and chopped

Directions:

1. Place all ingredients in a pot.
2. Close the lid and allow to boil for 15 minutes until the potatoes are soft.
3. Drain the potatoes and place in a food processor together with the dates.
4. Pulse until smooth.
5. Place in individual containers.
6. Put a label and store in the fridge.
7. Allow to thaw at room temperature before heating in the microwave oven.

Nutrition:

Calories: 619;

Carbs: 97.8g;

Protein: 4.8g;

Fat: 24.3g;

Sweet Potato Soup

Preparation Time: 10 minutes

Cooking Time: 30 minute

Servings: 4

Ingredients :

- Pepper and salt to taste
- 2 tbsp. thyme leaves
- Juice of half a lemon
- 1 tsp. ground cumin
- 2 cups mashed sweet potato
- 4 cups chicken stock
- 4 bell pepper, diced
- 1 onion, diced
- 1 tbsp. coconut oil

Directions:

1. On medium low fire, place a heavy bottomed pot and heat coconut oil.
2. Sauté peppers and onions for 5 minutes or until slightly soft.
3. Meanwhile, in a blender puree mashed sweet potatoes with 2 cups chicken stock. Pour into pot.

4. Add cumin and remaining chicken stock. Cover and bring to a boil.
5. Lower fire to a simmer and cook for 20 minutes or until peppers are tender.
6. Season with pepper, salt, thyme and lemon juice.
7. Serve while hot.

Nutrition:

Calories: 112;

Carbs: 17.5g;

Protein: 3.5g;

Fat: 4.6g

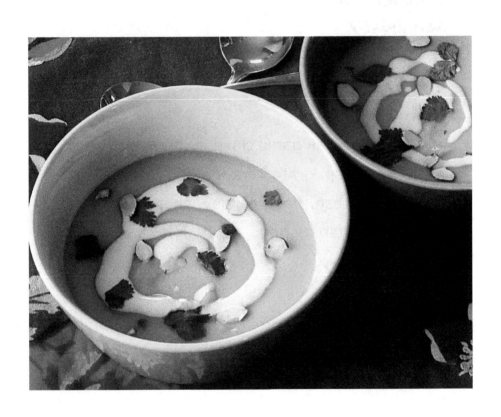

Sweet Potatoes Oven Fried

Preparation Time: 10 minutes

Cooking Time: 30 minute

Servings: 7

Ingredients :

- 1 small garlic clove, minced
- 1 tsp. grated orange rind
- 1 tbsp. fresh parsley, chopped finely
- ¼ tsp. pepper
- ¼ tsp. salt
- 1 tbsp. olive oil
- 4 medium sweet potatoes, peeled and sliced to ¼-inch thickness

Directions:

1. In a large bowl mix well pepper, salt, olive oil and sweet potatoes.
2. In a greased baking sheet, in a single layer arrange sweet potatoes.

3. Pop in a preheated 400oF oven and bake for 15 minutes, turnover potato slices and return to oven. Bake for another 15 minutes or until tender.
4. Meanwhile, mix well in a small bowl garlic, orange rind and parsley, sprinkle over cooked potato slices and serve.
5. You can store baked sweet potatoes in a lidded container and just microwave whenever you want to eat it. Do consume within 3 days.

Nutrition:

Calories: 176;

Carbs: 36.6g;

Protein: 2.5g;

Fat: 2.5g

Tasty Avocado Sauce over Zoodles

Preparation Time: 10 minutes

Cooking Time: 10 minute

Servings: 2

Ingredients :

- 1 zucchini peeled and spiralized into noodles
- 4 tbsp. pine nuts
- 2 tbsp. lemon juice
- 1 avocado peeled and pitted
- 12 sliced cherry tomatoes
- 1/3 cup water
- 1 1/4 cup basil
- Pepper and salt to taste

Directions:

1. Make the sauce in a blender by adding pine nuts, lemon juice, avocado, water, and basil.

Pulse until smooth and creamy. Season with pepper and salt to taste. Mix well.

2.   Place zoodles in salad bowl. Pour over avocado sauce and toss well to coat.

3.   Add cherry tomatoes, serve, and enjoy.

Nutrition:

Calories: 313;

Protein: 6.8g;

Carbs: 18.7g;

Fat: 26.8g

Tomato Basil Cauliflower Rice

Preparation Time: 5 minutes

Cooking Time: 10 minute

Servings: 4

Ingredients :

- Salt and pepper to taste
- Dried parsley for garnish
- ¼ cup tomato paste
- ½ tsp. garlic, minced
- ½ tsp. onion powder
- ½ tsp. marjoram
- 1 ½ tsp. dried basil
- 1 tsp. dried oregano
- 1 large head of cauliflower
- 1 tsp. oil

Directions:

1. Cut the cauliflower into florets and place in the food processor.
2. Pulse until it has a coarse consistency similar with rice. Set aside.
3. In a skillet, heat the oil and sauté the garlic and onion for three minutes. Add the rest of the ingredients. Cook for 8 minutes.

Nutrition:

Calories: 106;

Carbs: 15.1g;

Protein: 3.3g;

Fat: 5.0g

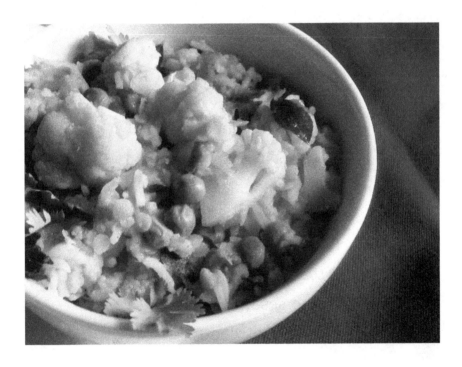

Vegan Sesame Tofu and Eggplants

Preparation Time: 10 minutes

Cooking Time: 20 minute

Servings: 4

Ingredients :

- 5 tbsp. olive oil
- 1-lb. firm tofu, sliced
- 3 tbsp. rice vinegar
- 2 tsp. Swerve sweetener
- 2 whole eggplants, sliced
- ¼ cup soy sauce
- Salt and pepper to taste
- 4 tbsp. toasted sesame oil
- ¼ cup sesame seeds
- 1 cup fresh cilantro, chopped

Directions:

1. Heat the oil in a pan for 2 minutes.

2. Pan fry the tofu for 3 minutes on each side.

3. Stir in the rice vinegar, sweetener, eggplants, and soy sauce. Season with salt and pepper to taste.

4. Cover and cook for 5 minutes on medium fire. Stir and continue cooking for another 5 minutes.

5. Toss in the sesame oil, sesame seeds, and cilantro.

6. Serve and enjoy.

Nutrition:

Calories: 616;

Carbs: 27.4g;

Protein: 23.9g;

Fat: 49.2g

Vegetarian Coconut Curry

Preparation Time: 10 minutes

Cooking Time: 30 minute

Servings: 4

Ingredients :

- 4 tbsp. coconut oil
- 1 medium onion, chopped
- 1 tsp. minced garlic
- 1 tsp. minced ginger
- 1 cup broccoli florets
- 2 cups fresh spinach leaves
- 2 tsp. fish sauce
- 1 tbsp. garam masala
- ½ cup coconut milk
- Salt and pepper to taste

Directions:

1. Heat oil in a pot.
2. Sauté the onion and garlic until fragrant, around 3 minutes.
3. Stir in the rest of the ingredients, except for spinach leaves.
4. Season with salt and pepper to taste.
5. Cover and cook on medium fire for 5 minutes.
6. Stir and add spinach leaves. Cover and cook for another 2 minutes.
7. Turn off fire and let it sit for two more minutes before serving.

Nutrition:

Calories: 210;

Carbs: 6.5g;

Protein: 2.1g;

Fat: 20.9g

Veggie Lo Mein

Preparation Time: 10 minutes

Cooking Time: 4 minute

Servings: 6

Ingredients :

- 2 tbsp. olive oil
- 5 cloves of garlic, minced
- 2-inch knob of ginger, grated
- 8 oz. mushrooms, sliced
- ½ lb. zucchini, spiralized
- 1 carrot, julienned
- 1 spring green onions, chopped
- 3 tbsp. coconut aminos
- Salt and pepper to taste
- 1 tbsp. sesame oil

Directions:

1. Heat the oil in a skillet and sauté the garlic and ginger until fragrant.

2. Stir in the mushrooms, zucchini, carrot, and green onions.
3. Season with coconut aminos, salt and pepper.
4. Close the lid and allow to simmer for 5 minutes.
5. Drizzle with sesame oil last.
6. Place in individual containers.
7. Put a label and store in the fridge.
8. Allow to thaw at room temperature before heating in the microwave oven.

Nutrition:

Calories 288;

Carbs: 48.7g;

Protein: 7.6g;

Fat: 11g;

Veggie Jamaican Stew

Preparation Time: 15 minutes

Cooking Time: 30 minute

Servings: 4

Ingredients :

- 1 tbsp. cilantro, chopped
- 1 tsp. salt
- 1 tsp. pepper
- 1 tbsp. lime juice
- 2 cups collard greens, sliced
- 3 cups carrots, cut into bite-sized chunks
- ½ yellow plantain, cut into bite-sized pieces
- 1 cup okra, cut into ½" pieces
- 2 cups potatoes, cut into bite-sized cubes
- 2 cups taro, cut into bite sized cubes
- 2 cups pumpkin, cut into bite sized cubes
- 2 cups water
- 2 cups coconut milk
- 2 bay leaves
- 3 green onions, white bottom removed
- ½ tsp. dried thyme
- ½ tsp. ground allspice
- 4 garlic cloves, minced

- 1 onion, chopped
- 1 tbsp. olive oil

Directions:

1. On medium fire, place a stockpot and heat oil. Sauté onions for 4 minutes or until translucent and soft. Add thyme, all spice and garlic. Sauté for a minute.
2. Pour in water and coconut milk and bring to a simmer. Add bay leaves and green onions.
3. Once simmering, slow fire to keep broth at a simmer and add taro and pumpkin. Cook for 5 minutes.
4. Add potatoes and cook for three minutes.
5. Add carrots, plantain and okra. Mix and cook for five minutes.
6. Then remove and fish for thyme sprigs, bay leaves and green onions and discard.
7. Add collard greens and cook for four minutes or until bright green and darker in color.
8. Turn off fire, add pepper, salt and lime juice to taste. Once it tastes good, mix well, transfer to a serving bowl, serve and enjoy.

Nutrition:

Calories: 531;

Carbs: 59.7g;

Protein: 8.3g;

Fat: 32.7g

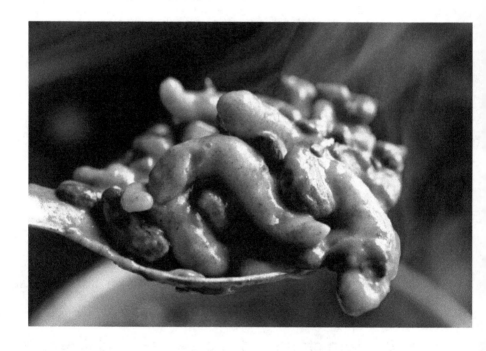

Vegetable Soup Moroccan Style

Preparation Time: 10 minutes

Cooking Time: 10 minute

Servings: 6

Ingredients :

- ½ tsp. pepper
- 1 tsp. salt
- 2 oz whole wheat orzo
- 1 large zucchini, peeled and cut into ¼-insh cubes
- 8 sprigs fresh cilantro, plus more leaves for garnish
- 12 sprigs flat leaf parsley, plus more for garnish
- A pinch of saffron threads
- 2 stalks celery leaves included, sliced thinly
- 2 carrots, diced
- 2 small turnips, peeled and diced
- 1 14-oz can diced tomatoes
- 6 cups water
- 1 lb. lamb stew meat, trimmed and cut into ½-inch cubes
- 2 tsp. ground turmeric
- 1 medium onion, diced finely

- 2 tbsp. extra virgin olive oil

Directions:

1. On medium high fire, place a large Dutch oven and heat oil.
2. Add turmeric and onion, stir fry for two minutes.
3. Add meat and sauté for 5 minutes.
4. Add saffron, celery, carrots, turnips, tomatoes and juice, and water.
5. With a kitchen string, tie cilantro and parsley sprigs together and into pot.
6. Cover and bring to a boil. Once boiling reduce fire to a simmer and continue to cook for 45 to 50 minutes or until meat is tender.
7. Once meat is tender, stir in zucchini. Cover and cook for 8 minutes.
8. Add orzo; cook for 10 minutes or until soft.
9. Remove and discard cilantro and parsley sprigs.
10. 1 Season with pepper and salt.
11. 1 Transfer to a serving bowl and garnish with cilantro and parsley leaves before serving.

Nutrition:

Calories: 268;

Carbs: 12.9g;

Protein: 28.1g;

Fat: 11.7g

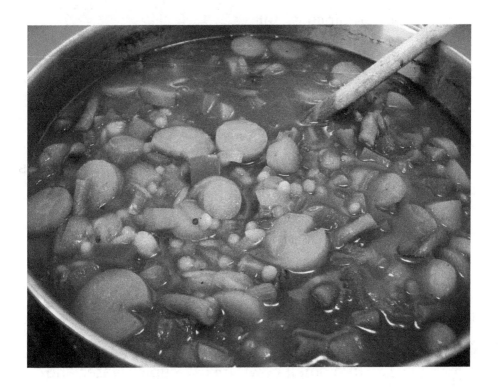

Veggie Ramen Miso Soup

Preparation Time: 5 minutes

Cooking Time: 20 minute

Servings: 1

Ingredients :

- 2 tsp. thinly sliced green onion
- A pinch of salt
- ½ tsp. shoyu
- 2 tbsp. mellow white miso
- 1 cup zucchini, cut into angel hair spirals
- ½ cup thinly sliced cremini mushrooms
- ½ medium carrot, cut into angel hair spirals
- 1/2 cup baby spinach leaves – optional
- 2 ¼ cups water
- ½ box of medium firm tofu, cut into ¼-inch cubes
- 1 hardboiled egg

Directions:

1. In a small bowl, mix ¼ cup of water and miso. Set aside.
2. In a small saucepan on medium high fire, bring to a boil 2 cups water, mushrooms, tofu and carrots. Add salt, shoyu and miso mixture. Allow to boil for 5 minutes. Remove

from fire and add green onion, zucchini and baby spinach leaves if using.

3.   Let soup stand for 5 minutes before transferring to individual bowls. Garnish with ½ of hardboiled egg per bowl, serve and enjoy.

Nutrition:

Calories: 335;

Carbs: 19.0g;

Protein: 30.6g;

Fat: 17.6g

Yummy Cauliflower Fritters

Preparation Time: 10 minutes

Cooking Time: 15 minute

Servings: 6

Ingredients :

- 1 large cauliflower head, cut into florets
- 2 eggs, beaten
- ½ tsp. turmeric
- ½ tsp. salt
- ¼ tsp. black pepper
- 6 tbsp. coconut oil

Directions:

1. Place the cauliflower florets in a pot with water.
2. Bring to a boil and drain once cooked.
3. Place the cauliflower, eggs, turmeric, salt, and pepper into the food processor.
4. Pulse until the mixture becomes coarse.
5. Transfer into a bowl. Using your hands, form six small flattened balls and place in the fridge for at least 1 hour until the mixture hardens.
6. Heat the oil in a skillet and fry the cauliflower patties for 3 minutes on each side

7. Place in individual containers.

8. Put a label and store in the fridge.

9. Allow to thaw at room temperature before heating in the microwave oven.

Nutrition:

Calories 157;

Carbs: 2.8g;

Protein: 3.9g;

Fat: 15.3g;

Fiber: 0.9g

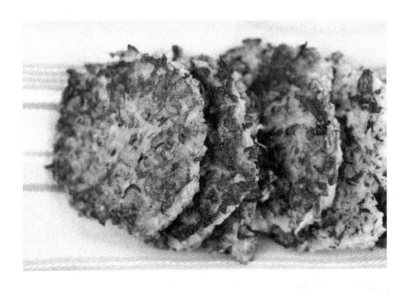

Zucchini Garlic Fries

Preparation Time: 15 minutes

Cooking Time: 20 minute

Servings: 6

Ingredients :

- ¼ tsp. garlic powder
- ½ cup almond flour
- 2 large egg whites, beaten
- 3 medium zucchinis, sliced into fry sticks
- Salt and pepper to taste

Directions:

1. Preheat oven to 400°F.
2. Mix all ingredients in a bowl until the zucchini fries are well coated.
3. Place fries on cookie sheet and spread evenly.
4. Put in oven and cook for 20 minutes.
5. Halfway through cooking time, stir fries.

Nutrition:

Calories: 11;

Carbs: 1.1g;

Protein: 1.5g;

Fat: 0.1g

Zucchini Pasta with Mango-Kiwi Sauce

Preparation Time: 5 minutes

Cooking Time: 20 minute

Servings: 2

Ingredients :

- 1 tsp. dried herbs – optional
- ½ Cup Raw Kale leaves, shredded
- 2 small dried figs
- 3 medjool dates
- 4 medium kiwis
- 2 big mangos, seed discarded
- 2 cup zucchini, spiralized
- ¼ cup roasted cashew

Directions:

1. On a salad bowl, place kale then topped with zucchini noodles and sprinkle with dried herbs. Set aside.

2. In a food processor, grind to a powder the cashews. Add figs, dates, kiwis and mangoes then puree to a smooth consistency.

3. Pour over zucchini pasta, serve and enjoy.

Nutrition:

Calories: 530;

Carbs: 95.4g;

Protein: 8.0g;

Fat: 18.5g

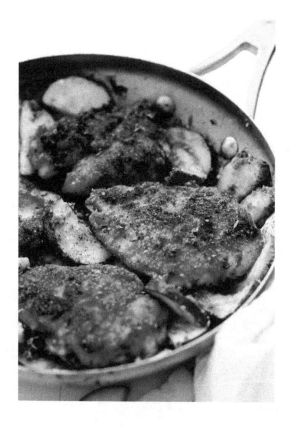

Quinoa with Almonds and Cranberries
Preparation Time: 10 minutes

Cooking Time: 15 minute

Servings: 4

Ingredients :

- 2 cups cooked quinoa
- 1/3 tsp. cranberries or currants
- ¼ cup sliced almonds
- 2 garlic cloves, minced
- 1¼ tsp. salt
- ½ tsp. ground cumin
- ½ tsp. turmeric
- ¼ tsp. ground cinnamon
- ¼ tsp. freshly ground black pepper

Directions:

1. In a large bowl, toss the quinoa, cranberries, almonds, garlic, salt, cumin, turmeric, cinnamon, and pepper and stir to combine. Enjoy alone or with roasted cauliflower.

Nutrition:

Calories: 430;

Carbs: 65.4g;

Protein: 8.0g;

Fat: 15.5g

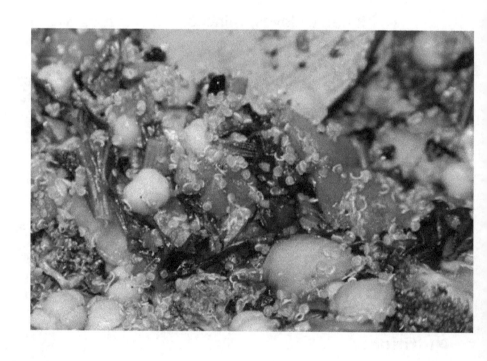